Reflection for Paramed and Beyd

CW00516634

By
Karen Gubbins, Sue Lillyman and Tony Ghaye

1

Edition 2

Published in 2016 by New Vista Publications
Part of Reflective Learning-International
Overton Business Centre
Maisemore
Gloucester
GL2 8HR
England

www.rl-international.com

Authors: Karen Gubbins, Sue Lillyman and Tony Ghaye
Cover Design: Karen Gubbins
Book Design and Formatting: Karen Gubbins, Sue Lillyman and Tony Ghaye

Contents

About the authors

Karen Gubbins MSc, BSc (Hons), DipHE in Paramedic Studies, PG Cert.

Karen Gubbins started a career in healthcare at the Dental Hospital in Birmingham in 1992. She then moved to the West Midlands Ambulance Service NHS Trust becoming a Trainee Paramedic in 1996, and qualified as a Paramedic in 1998. She worked at a number of stations within the West Midlands, gaining promotion to first line manager, and then worked as a training officer for a number of years within an ambulance service. In 2007, she moved into higher education and commenced work with the University of Worcester. She is currently a senior lecturer teaching on the Foundation Degree in Paramedic Science. She studied for a BSc (Hons), PGCert and MSc all at the University of Worcester. She is still practicing as a Paramedic and has a special interest in paramedic reflection.

Sue Lillyman MA (ed), BSc (Nursing), RGN, RM, DPSN, PGCE, (FAHE), RNT.

Sue is a qualified Registered General Nurse and Midwife. She has clinical experience in various areas of nursing including: intensive care, gynaecology and care of the elderly, rehabilitation, acute medicine and tropical medicine. Sue entered nurse education in 1989. She is currently working at the University of Worcester where she continues to have a passion for developing and enhancing clinical practice through reflection. She is well published in the area and currently involved in introducing and working with colleagues in East Africa to implement reflection and reflective practice into the nursing curricula there.

Tony Ghaye Cert.Ed, BEd. (Hons) MA, PhD. FRSA

In Tony's working life he has been fortunate in being able to work with and learn from a very wide range of professionals, including nurses, midwives, health visitors, GPs, social workers, police and probation officers, therapists of various kinds, osteopaths, sports coaches and school teachers. Tony has also experienced the privilege and challenge of working with individuals and communities in the Third World and in emerging nations in East Africa. All this experience has energised his commitment to inter-professional learning and multidisciplinary working to help to improve what we do with and for others. He sees learning through the practices of reflection as a central part of his work on quality of life issues, personal development and service improvement. He is the Director of Reflective Learning-International (www.rl-international.com) and founder and editor-in-chief of the multi-professional international journal published by Routledge Taylor and Francis called, 'Reflective Practice: International and Multidisciplinary Perspectives'.

Acknowledgements

We would like to acknowledge all our colleagues and students for their support and encouragement in the preparation of this book.

The authors would especially like to thank paramedic Kim Griffin for her time, proof reading and comments that have helped to make this publication accessible and useful.

Our thanks also go to Jules Holland for her help with this publication.

Introduction

This book is designed to help you during your education to become a paramedic, and once qualified as a paramedic, to develop reflective skills in order to maintain and develop as a professional. It is designed to provide you with strategies and guide you through the process of reflection and how to develop as a reflective practitioner/paramedic. Part of becoming a reflective paramedic is also to gain knowledge in relation to reflection as well as enhance your critical and creative thinking skills. The book will provide you with a selection of reflective tools that can assist you to produce clinical and reflective records, journals and critical incidents that you can use as evidence of your development in a written format in line with the College of Paramedics (2015) and Health and Care Professional Council's (2014) requirements for your continuing professional development (CPD) to remain on the register. And for those who work in the National Health Service it will also provide guidance on achieving your evidence for your appraisal and meeting your Knowledge and Skills Framework (KSF) (DoH 2004) requirements.

This book will enable you to gain a better understanding of who you are, what you do, what your strengths are and how you can continue to improve your work. By using the different practices of reflection, and, by becoming a reflective paramedic we hope you will develop your competencies to deliver and manage safe and high quality care. The following six key ideas of reflection outline aims that you may aspire to achieve during the reflective process.

The Six key ideas of reflection:

1. Reflective practices help us understand the links between what we do (our work) and how we might improve our effectiveness (by developing our practice). For example, reflective practices help us understand the importance of practicing safely and provide ideas and options for developing our work. Reflection is therefore linked to practice. Through reflection we can develop new insights and understandings that help us to improve our actions. Reflective practices are aimed at improving what you are really doing.

2. Reflective practices also help us understand the links between feeling, thinking and doing. How we feel effects how we think. This effects what we actually do. It is important to join these three things up if you want to get better at your work.

3. Reflection is often described as 'structured' or organised thinking. So what might you think about? Maybe about your feelings because your work is influenced by emotions (e.g. how you feel, how your patients feel and how your colleagues are feeling). Your work is also guided by what you think and the context in which you practice.

4. We can understand our practice by looking backwards. Looking back on your experiences and learning from them is important. But reflecting on the past can be limited by what we can remember and by what has happened. It is also important to reflect on the here-and-now. To reflect not only on what has happened or what we would like to happen, but with what's happening now. There are many kinds of reflection which we explore in this book.

5. It is very important to use reflection to help you identify, develop and amplify what you can do, not just what you cannot do. It is very important to reflect on your strengths. It is not always necessary to focus first on your problems and the difficult aspects of the situation/experience you are thinking about. What would it cost you to begin by looking at the successful aspects of the experience first and to devote your energy to amplifying what went well? This might help you get rid of the negative feelings you may associate with reflection.

6. Reflection can be triggered by many things. One is a question. It is important to know the difference between a deficit-based question (e.g. what went wrong) and a strengths-based question (e.g. what went well?). The latter can be called a 'positive question'. Strengths-based reflective practices draw upon the power of the positive question.

Reflection is a skilled practice. It uses experience, knowledge and inquiry processes to increase our ability to intervene, interpret, and act positively on successes, problems, and significant paramedic related issues. The use of particular reflective activities can reveal new insights and understandings about who we are and what we do. These practices can also reveal options, possibilities and avenues for positive and sustainable paramedic action. In this sense then, one outcome of reflection is the creation of new, useable and hopefully, better knowledge. The kind of knowledge that will help you practice in a safe, ethical and efficient way.

EXPERIENCE plays a central role in learning through reflection. We can understand 'experience' as something that is lived, felt, reconstructed, reinterpreted, and understood. If we take a positive view on this, reflecting on particular experiences, enables us to make sense and meaning of our encounters with others. These may be patients, clients, carers, family members, colleagues and so on. Sense and meaning are built-up, or 'constructed', through the use of reflective practices. This is very different from simply thinking that we can discover meaning, already nicely packaged-up and 'out there', somewhere in the workplace. We cannot always get useful knowledge off a library shelf! We have to 'make' it ourselves.

These encounters and experiences occur in a **CONTEXT**. There are different ways to describe a context. For example it might be a private or a public context, a current or an historical context, a home or a clinical context. Each context has social and often political aspects to it. Sometimes these aspects are visible. At other times these aspects are rather more tricky to 'see'. In most contexts there are people doing things like working, playing, making decisions and engaging in many other kinds of conscious and intentional activities. All these activities require a level of motivation. More generally a context can be regarded as a space for particular actions. In this book we are talking about contexts in which healthcare is learned, managed or delivered.

In many workplaces, the dominant **CULTURE** is one of doing, with little time for reflection and therefore, for workplace learning. In general, *cultures of doing* can be described in many ways. For example as high or low performing. They can be characterised by busyness, pressure, targets and deadlines. They can be described as workplace *cultures of appreciation*, where everyone feels valued and respected, or as *cultures of blame* where the languages of 'not being good enough', of poor performance, of inefficiency, and 'it's not my fault' dominate.

So when you reflect on your work, it is important to think about;

- Pleasure - how you feel about yourself and what you do

- Purpose - being able to engage in something you feel is worthwhile

- Fulfillment - achieving your goals and knowing you are doing well

Chapter 1

Reflection and reflective practice for Continuing Professional Development and course work

Introduction

The process of reflection and reflective practice has been identified as crucial to the development of paramedics. This has been included within all training programmes for paramedics and following registration by the College of Paramedics which included the use of reflection in their requirements for CPD for all paramedics. It is also included within the Health and Care Professions Councils (2014) CPD framework that allows you to remain registered as a paramedic once qualified.

For those paramedics that work within the NHS there is s further requirement for reflection and development for the Knowledge and Skills Framework (DoH 2004). This framework focuses on the application of knowledge and skills. It requires you to demonstrate the application of your knowledge to your practice. This application can be achieved through the process of reflection.

Reflection then is not just part of your training course but it will be a skill that is required in your role as a paramedic and throughout your career.

Origins of reflection

Reflection was a concept first written about by an educational theorist John Dewey in 1933. Dewey (1933) believed that reflective thinking often arose out of situations of doubt, hesitation, perplexity and/or mental difficulty. These situations he suggested prompted the person to search, hunt, or inquire, in order to find material that would resolve doubt and settle or dispose the perplexity. Dewey (1933) acknowledged the importance of past experiences for reflection and argued that ideas and suggestions are dependent on one's past experiences as they do not arise out of nothing.

Donald Schön (1987), an American philosopher and musician, also wrote extensively on reflection identifying two approaches of reflection-on-action and reflection-in-action. His approach is discussed in more detail in chapter 2.

Schön followed the work of Dewey in the 1970's -1990's and introduced such concepts as 'the learning society' (Schön 1973), 'double loop learning' (Argyris and Schön 1974) and the 'ability to think on your feet' (Schön 1983). He also suggested that change was a fundamental feature of modern society and that there was a need for professionals to develop social systems to cope, adapt and be flexible to change whilst at the same time maintaining their identity.

In their double loop learning theory, Argyris and Schön (1974) also introduced the concept of mental mind maps that people use rather than basing their practice on theories.

Kolb (1984) developed this further when he talked about 'experiential learning' with a further development from Finger and Asun (2000) who talked about abstract conceptualisation, this they suggested is analysing and working from the analysis.

Since these original writers there has been a lot of interest and literature within the past few decades. Reflection and reflective practice is now being incorporated into many educational programmes and as part of the continuing professional development for the majority of health care professionals including paramedics, education, social care, police, business and many other professional groups.

You can read more about these theorists and their critics in the literature. In this book we are reviewing how reflection and reflective practice is useful to you as a paramedic. This background helps to place development of reflection and how it was introduced into professional practice.

What is reflection?

Taylor (2006 pg 17) quoted Plato as saying 'the un-reflected life is not worth living'. To reflect then must have some meaning to our lives and practice and not be seen as a waste of time and effort. Reflection is a process that helps you to develop the ability to examine your own actions, thoughts, feelings and think purposefully about your clinical practice in order to gain new insights, ideas and understanding (Newell 1992 and Haddock, 1997). According to Kim and Lee (2002), reflection refers to active, intellectual thinking for monitoring your practice and seeking new opportunities to learn how to do new and better things. This suggests that reflection is more than simply thinking about what you do, but is an active process resulting in learning (Cooney 1999).

What is reflective practice?

Reflective practice has been included within many curricula for health care professionals, and more recently for paramedics. It is referred to within clinical practice and literature, yet, the terminology is not always fully understood by practitioners (Powell 1989 and Gelter 2003). In the early 1990's there was much debate within literature as to the definition, value and implementation of the role of reflective practitioners within the clinical field (Jarvis 1992). This led, in many situations, to practitioners becoming more confused as to its relevance and its value to their individual clinical practice.

Today we have a clearer picture and view reflective practice as what Jarvis (1992) called 'thoughtful practice'. Jarvis (1992) suggests that our actions are based on previous learning, theory and the continuing monitoring of our actions in practice. Being a reflective practitioner also means that you, as the paramedic, can learn through your practice and that you can justify your practice through reflecting on your experiences and applying theories to that practice (Ghaye and Lillyman 2006). It is a process that helps you maintain and develop as a practitioner and keep up to date within this ever changing world.

Becoming competent reflective practitioners/paramedics

Your course will provide you with the skills to be a competent paramedic practitioner at the point of qualifying. However to continuously develop throughout your career; especially once you have qualified you need to be learning how to be a self-directed learner and competent reflective paramedic practitioner.

As a paramedic you need to examine the rationale that underpins what you may initially take for granted as right natural practice situations. You are also asked to question your own views of and reaction to your practice in order to become that competent reflective paramedic practitioner.

You also need to develop a desire to synthesise diverse ideas, to make sense out of nonsense, and apply information in an inspired direction to your work. To question what you are doing and why you are doing it that way. This is not an easy option and to truly become a reflective paramedic Dewey (1933) suggested that you need to be open minded, take responsibility for your practice and be wholehearted to its approach.

Becoming a reflective paramedic will help you to work through your fears and insecurities and therefore give you the courage to analyse and evaluate your practice situations, society, patients as well as yourself.

Using reflection for course work

As stated earlier, all training courses for the role of paramedic will include the use and development of reflection. Many modules ask you to write a reflective account and/or record or maintain a professional learning journal as part of the course work. All these processes assist you to develop those reflective skills that help you to become and develop as a competent reflective paramedic throughout your career. Writing such an essay can be a daunting process at the start. However there are many models of reflection that can help you frame the essay such as Gibbs (1988), Johns (2004), Atkins and Murphy (1994), Mezirow (1981) to name a few. These are discussed further in chapter 3.

By using a model of your choice you can frame the essay. The tendency for reflective essays at first to be descriptive and can result in lower marks at diploma level and above course work. You should avoid taking too much time over the description of the experience and concentrate on that critical analysis, evaluation and learning in order to produce a good academic assignment. See example 5. Concentrating on the analysis, evaluation and learning will again further develop those reflective skills for practice.

One of the issues with reflection is that it can become very negative and only focus on what has gone wrong in your practice. Models like Atkins and Murphy (1994) start by asking you to identify 'awareness of uncomfortable feelings and thoughts'. However you need to remember that we can also develop and learn from things that went well. We will continue to emphasis this throughout this book. Reflection is not a tool to beat ourselves with when things go wrong, but a tool that can help us to develop our practice. We are not saying that when things do not go as expected we should not reflect on those, as we always want to improve our practice, but we should equally celebrate the strengths and good practice as we can also learn from them.

This positive approach is referred to as *Appreciative reflection.* This approach was introduced by Ghaye et al (2008), who suggests that we review the positive aspects of our practice before we work on the challenging areas. They suggest it is about building on strengths. This approach is discussed further in chapter 3.

Reflection for Continuing Professional Development

One of the main aims of using reflection and this approach is that you can also develop the skills to become a self-directed learner and a competent reflective paramedic throughout your career. Ramnarayan & Hande (2005) highlighted that self-directed learning as essential to meet the challenges in today's changing health care environment.

Becoming a self-directed learner

As part of your professional development, and in order to remain on the Health and Care Professions Councils register to practice as a paramedic, you are expected to become a self-directed learner and continuously engage in the acquisition and application of knowledge and skills (Fischer & Scharff 1998). Chene (1983) suggest the following three elements that characterise self-directed learners:

 ❖ independence, ability to make choices

 ❖ the capacity to articulate the norms

 ❖ the limits of a learning activity

Becoming a critical thinker

Critical thinking is also an important process in becoming a reflective paramedic. Through thinking critically you can gain a broader outlook on your practice, become creative in relation to finding solutions and the identification of multiple pathways needed for successful quality improvement initiatives (Simpson & Courteney 2000).

Being a critical thinker, according to Ghaye et al (2008), involves probing, questioning and putting ideas under pressure which will assist you in clinical decision making and in making clinical judgements. Critical thinking is increasingly being recognised as the cognitive engine driving the process of knowledge development and professional judgement in a wide variety of professional practice fields (Facione & Facione 1996).

Rubenfeld and Scheffer (1999) believed that critical thinking also includes confidence, contextual perspective, creativity, flexibility, inquisitiveness, intellectual integrity, intuition, open-mindedness, perseverance and 'reflection'. Yahiro and Saylor (1994) defined it as reflective and reasoned thinking about problems without one solution. Additionally Facione and

Facione (1996) defined critical thinking as purposeful, self-regulatory judgement, an interactive, and reflective reasoning process of making a judgement about what to believe or to do. Chafee (1994) goes onto suggest that critical thinking opens the door to new perspectives about the world, fosters self-confidence, and encourages life-long learning. All these aspects are important for your professional development as a paramedic.

Maintaining records for your continuing professional development

There are a variety of ways, models and frameworks that can be used to record a reflective account either for an assignment or as part of your professional portfolio. These include the use of critical incidents, journals, mind maps, diaries and profiles of evidence. Each is discussed in more detail in the following chapter.

In order to provide evidence that you are reflecting and developing your practice you need to record your reflection within your portfolio. This is usually saved in a written form and filed. It can then be used, by you, in your annual appraisal to provide evidence of completing the KSF requirements if you work within the NHS, or for the HPC who randomly select paramedic's portfolios for review. You can also use it within an interview to demonstrate your reflection/development of your practice providing examples from your practice.

For the paramedic, the Health and Care Professions Council advocate the use of on-line or written portfolio.

The College of Paramedics (2015) state that the profile should include:

- Personal details
- Contents page
- Curriculum Vitae
- Professional practice
- Job description
- Personal development plan
- Reflections and articles
- Consent forms
- Certificates
- Record of clinical experience
- Competence and practice outcomes
- Essential supplement information
- Evidence matrix.

They also offer an on line version available at https://www.collegeofparamedics.co.uk/ that you can access and complete on line as a paramedic.

The Health and Care Professions Council completes random sampling of the profiles that are submitted for review on request at re-registration. You should therefore keep it up to date at all times.

Chapter 2

Strategies and activities in becoming a reflective paramedic

Introduction

In this chapter we explore some of the supporting strategies and activities you can use to assist you with reflection. It will suggest, and give examples of, practical approaches to developing a reflective culture and becoming a reflective practitioner.

Learning event or critical incident

Before you can start to reflect you need something to reflect on. John Flannagan (1954) first described the use of a 'critical incident' and Tripp in 1993 developed the work further. They reviewed how practice is changed and developed through critical thinking and analysing practice. The term 'critical incident' can be misleading as it implies, by its name, that this is a major negative event or experience. However in health care when we talk about critical incidents, we can use the term 'learning event/experience' or 'significant event'. They do not need to be major, or for that matter negative, they are an experience that has made you stop and think, either it has been demanding, different, new or made you draw on past experience or theory. This event could be something that surprised you in your reactions or thoughts, challenged you or reinforced your practice (Ghaye and Lillyman 2006). Although we often use our own experiences to reflect on there is a place to learn from observing other paramedics and listening to others through storytelling and using narratives (Spouse 2003 and Lillyman et al 2011).

Reflection should always be moving our practice or informing the practice we do in some way. Although every event will not be life changing for you each builds on the last to make you the paramedic you are or want to become.

The time line for the event/experience can vary; it might take a second or a few minutes to a month or over a period of years. This can also be seen in Schön's (1983, 1987) work where he talks about reflection-on-action.

Reflection-on-action, Schön (1987) describes, is looking back at your practice. Indentifying what happened, why it happened, what you could do to improve, justify or maintain in that practice. He also referred to reflection-in-action that he suggests thinking about your practice as you are working through it. Here you can draw on those previous experiences that now inform that practice.

However there is not only the looking back at practice and thinking about current practice, there is what Van Manen (1977) described as anticipated reflection. For example what goes through your mind when you received your first 999 call, as you plan about how you will react before the call even comes through, what you might do and what you might say, how you might react is often all rehearsed through your thoughts before you even receive that call.

Each event you live through can be a catalyst for reflection however there is a danger of over reflecting.

Through reflection you can learn about your practice, plan out your practice before you encounter events and identify how to develop your future practice.

Reflective tools

Learning journal/diary/learning log

The use of written or oral records of the events and learning can be useful when demonstrating how you have learnt or applied theory to your practice. These can be in the form of learning journals, diary, learning logs, video diaries or taped voice diaries. These recordings can be used as 'aid memoir' for when you want to write a more formal reflection in your essay or Continuing Professional Development Portfolio. These recordings and writings are confidential and should not be handed in as part of your course work. From these however you can produce a more formal reflection that can then be produced for an assignment for your course or as a written reflection for a professional portfolio to demonstrate continuing professional development following registration (Lake 2001; Ghaye & Lillyman 2006).

Mind maps

Another form of recording reflections maybe through drawing mind maps. These are drawing in the forms of maps that connect one thought or topic to another, and help you organise and analyse information (Conceicao and Taylor 2007). They can be used as a focus for discussion with your critical friend. Bulman and Schutz (2004) suggest several benefits from concept mapping which include: facilitating decision making processes and revealing the tacit knowledge that underpins practice. Germann and Young-soo (2001) also suggest that they help to establish connections between bits of information, identify relationships between ideas, processes, actions and between new and old information. Mind maps can be drawn by hand, or created using computer software, depending upon your preference (see figure 2.1).

Figure 2.1 An example of a basic mind map

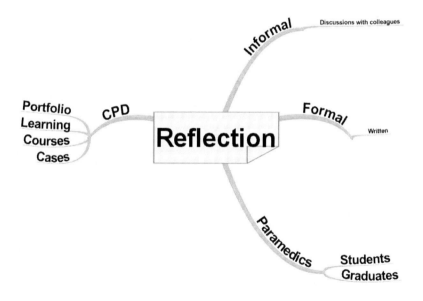

R-Card Learning

Another tool that can be used to record your reflections and can assist with committing your thoughts and reflections to writing are the R-Card Learning record sheets. The R-Card (see Fig. 2.2), has two sides to it. These cards are to use and record your reflection whilst in practice. Your reflections-in-action are entered on the small R-Card (the size of a credit card) which can be easily carried in your pocket. The R-Cards help you develop your competency in 5 areas and only take a minute to complete. They encourage fast and focused reflection, in the workplace. After completion, and when you have time away from work you can you can complete an R-Learning Record sheet (see Fig. 2.3) which will enrich and anchor your learning. On the follow-up R-Learning Record sheet (Figure 2.4), then you can use the R-Card to think again, and in more detail about: what the situation was, what your experience and motivation were, your personal values and confidence. On the R-Learning Record sheet you are encouraged to develop a personal action plan. The Record Sheets are completed away from practice. This is reflection-on-practice. You are required to answer the question, what have you learnt from the incident? From this you can identify an agreed action plan that has been discussed with your tutor, mentor or critical friend.

The R-Learning Cards can assist you in recording your learning and the first side can be completed within the work place (reflection-in-action). You can tick the relevant boxes to identify what type of experience you are focusing on. You can see from the completed examples in chapter 5 that you might tick more than one box for an experience. For example if you are taking a patients full history you might have to make a decision as to the type of questions are appropriate, therefore there will be some communication with the patient or other family/carers in relation to the questions and you might have to make some judgements about the mental capacity of your patient.

Once you have decided which aspects the incident involves then you can write a short description of the incident or learning event. This is short and quick to complete and can be used to remind you of the event rather than writing a full account or essay at the time.

Figure 2.2

R-Card – Side 1

Date:	Place of incident:
	(Do not give patients address, you only need to say if it was for example, at their home, or in a public space
Competency (tick relevant boxes) ETHICAL PERCEPTIONS ☐ JUDGEMENT ☐ TEAMWORKING ☐ DECISION MAKING ☐ COMMUNICATION ☐	

R-Card – Side 2

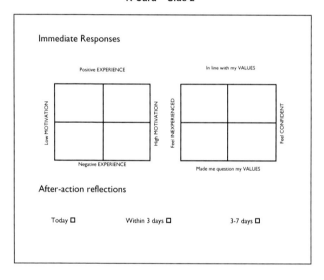

An explanation of side 2 of the R-Card is given below.

Positive/Negative EXPERIENCES	What did it feel like observing or participating in this event?
High /Low MOTIVATION	How far do you feel motivated to change, improve or maintain what you observed or participated in?

Once completed you complete in the values and confidence box. These are explained on the next page.

In line with, or made me question my VALUES	Your values affect how you feel and guide what you do. Has the event made you question your values? Confirmed them?
Feel CONFIDENT or feel inexperienced	How far did you feel confident or feel inexperienced in this situation?

Figure 2.3   R-LEARNING RECORD SHEET - SIDE 1

R-LEARNING RECORD SHEET - SIDE 1

1. **Event/Incident**:

2. Look at your **EXPERIENCE/MOTIVATION**, what is the most important thing you are learning?

3. Look at your **VALUES/CONFIDENCE**, what is the most important thing you are learning?

4. My **priority for action** is ...

Figure 2.4   **R-LEARNING RECORD SHEET – SIDE 2**

REFLECTIVE NOTES

State what you feel you have learned from using your R-Card/s:

Following discussion, what is your agreed action plan:

Following discussion this must be signed by either your mentor/facilitator or tutor:

Signature .... Date ....

Following the completion of the R-Card and R-Learning Record Sheet, you are required to complete the last box on the page of the Record Sheet which asks for an action plan (figure 2.4). This should be discussed with other colleagues, your mentor or supervisor.

Before completing the R-Learning Record Sheet, it is suggested that you take time away from the event and use this to reflect after the event and maybe discuss it with a critical friend (as noted below), or with peers to gain some collective wisdom on the event. This process aids the recollection of the event, includes some reflection in and on action and acts as evidence of learning. At a later date this can be developed further, if required for course content. For example, the incident can be developed using a reflective model to complete an essay or further analysis to demonstrate how theory relates to practice or how theory is generated from practice.

A Critical Friend

A critical friend is a trusted and experienced colleague, peer or mentor who can listen and advise you on your reflections. They can help to apply the theory into your practice and gain what Ghaye et al (2008) refers to as '*collective wisdom'*. With the critical friend you will need to engage in a *critical conversation*. This is more than a chat over a drink or a social event. It is very much part of the reflective learning process. By identifying a specific time and place it is easier to focus on the event in question than to just exchange stories. The conversation requires some structure and may include the following:

❖ Looking back and going over significant events

❖ Sharing your incident or journal entry

❖ Celebrating your success

❖ Indentifying where you need to improve your practice

❖ Deciding how you can improve and move your practice forward

❖ Agreeing with your critical friend what your next step or action plan might be

❖ Identifying a date for the next meeting

(Adapted from Ghaye and Lillyman 2006)

Support

Although many practitioners reflect on their own, Johns (1994) suggests that practitioners should have some supervision and/or coaching through the process. This can be in the form of a critical friend, as noted above, or support from a supervisor in practice and/or tutor/mentor. As you start to engage in reflection you may require guidance and support through the process. Knowing where to start, where to go with the content of reflection and when to stop can be developed further in the conversations with others. Too much reflection can result in damaging your self-esteem and your confidence, and lead to inaction. Appropriate guidance can prevent this from occurring.

Through this reflection you are expected to develop your practice and become autonomous practitioners at the end of your training, and develop your expertise in various aspects throughout your career.

Summary

If you are to become a reflective paramedic then you need to take responsibility for your development. This process begins as soon as you commence your initial training and develops throughout your career.

The following chapter identifies some reflective models and approaches that can be used to develop these skills further.

Chapter 3

Models and approaches to reflection

To facilitate your reflective skills, different models for reflection have been developed and can be used to guide you. A selection of models are offered within this chapter, although there are many more within the literature. We use the term 'model' generally to refer to a structured facilitative process. A model may be cyclical, be characterised by questions, levels and so on. In this chapter the 'models' we have chosen include Ghaye et al's (2008) appreciative approach, Gibbs's reflective cycle (1988), Mezirow's (1981) level of reflexivity and John's model (1994) of structured reflection. Many authors such as Bulman & Schutz (2004), Ghaye & Lillyman (2006), Johns (2006), Taylor (2006) and Quinn's & Hughes (2007) have acknowledged the contributions of reflective models and their impact on current practice. Also since reflection is not a static process, but a dynamic one, it is appropriate to include a framework that is action-oriented in its approach.

So what are models for? They;

❖ *'Help you to learn from your experience because they are practitioner focused. As part of this process they help you to develop a greater sense of personal-professional biography and history.*

❖ *Engage you in the process of knowledge creation by helping you to move from tacit knowing to more conscious and explicit knowing.*

❖ *Help you to overcome professional inertia by asking you to look at what you do, your taken-for-granted clinical worlds and that which is atypical, 'critical' and professionally significant.*

❖ *Tend to add more meaning and ascribe new and relevant meaning to your clinical practice through reflexive conversations with clinical situations. In this sense they enhance meaningful dialogue.*

❖ *Have some significance for future personal and sometimes collective future action.*

❖ *Celebrate the role of human agency'.*

(Ghaye and Lillyman 2006 pg 16)

The models can be grouped into different types. As stated previously, they can assist you to make learning from their experiences more explicit and provide a framework for you to work through.

Appreciative approach

This approach, developed by Ghaye et al (2008), introduces the notion of the positive and appreciative forms of reflection. As stated previously one of the dangers of reflection is that it can lead you to only reflect on negative aspects of care and practice. The appreciative approach very much focuses on the positive and allows you to build on incidents and experiences that have gone well. In this model Ghaye and his colleagues suggest that you as the learner, or practitioner, move away from 'problems' to a 'strength' based approach. However they note it is not a check list of activities but you must incorporate some personal reflection from your practice. The following questions initiate this appreciative process:

1. What's currently working well and why?
2. What needs changing and how?
3. What are you/we learning and so what do we need to do next?
4. Where do you/we go from here and what are the implications for improving your/our future clinical and managerial action and organisational culture/s?

The stages in this approach include the following:

- Developing appreciations
- Re-framing experience
- Building collective wisdom
- Achieving and moving forward

In more detail these mean:

❖ To **appreciate** the strengths and limitations, the gifts and talents of the practitioner and to appreciate their feeling in relation to the situation.

- ❖ To **re-frame** experience so that they can see things differently, in new and creative ways. This might include viewing alternative strategies.

- ❖ To **build collective wisdom** about their practice through reflective conversations, with each other. Reflective learning is not only about 'fixing' and getting rid of 'problems'. It is about identifying strengths, talking about success and knowing how to amplify (get more of) this. It is about building on strengths, not just about trying to get rid of problems.

- ❖ To put what the practitioner has learned through reflection, to good use to help **move practice** (and policy) **forward**.

The process is shown in Figure 3.1.

Figure 3.1   Ghaye et al's (2008) appreciative reflective process

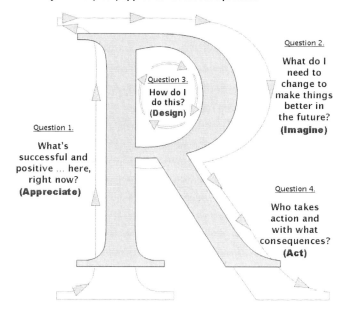

Question 2.

What do I need to change to make things better in the future?
(Imagine)

Question 3.

How do I do this?
(Design)

Question 1.

What's successful and positive … here, right now?
(Appreciate)

Question 4.

Who takes action and with what consequences?
(Act)

Structured Models

Models using cue questions

There are a number of structured models that use cue questions, including Johns (1994), Smyth (1991) and Burton (2000).

We include Johns (1994) model, a nurse by background, who produced a structured approach that was aimed at health care workers where he uses a series of cue questions to guide you through the process of reflection. He groups the questions in five ways:

- Description
- Reflection
- Influencing factors
- Alternative strategies
- Learning

For each he includes some cue, or trigger questions, to navigate you through the process. These are based on the 'what', 'why' and 'how'. See Figure 3.2.

Smyth (1991) had a similar model where he refers to 'moments' which were also linked to the following questions:

- Describe: what do I do?
- Inform: what does this description mean?
- Confront: how did I come to be like this?
- Reconstruct: how might I do things differently?

Smyth also offers a series of further probing questions to identify the underlying assumptions of practice.

Burton (2000) bases their model on three questions: what?, so what? and, now what? In order to achieve these there are guided questions which include:

Figure 3.2   Johns model of reflection

The following cues are offered to help practitioner's access, make sense of, and learn through experience.

1. Description
  1.1   Write a description of the experience
  1.2   What are the key issues within this description that I need to pay attention to?

2 Reflection
  2.1   What was I trying to achieve?
  2.2   Why did I act as I did?
  2.3   What are the consequences of my actions?
            For the patient and family?
            For myself?
            For the people I work with?
  2.4   How did I feel about this experience when it was happening?
  2.5   How did the patient feel about it?
  2.6   How do I know how the patient felt about it?

3 Influencing factors
  3.1   What internal factors influenced my decision-making and actions?
  3.2   What external factors influenced my decision-making and actions?
  3..3   What sources of knowledge did or should have influenced my decision-making and actions?

4 Alternative strategies
  4.1   Could I have dealt better with the situation?
  4.2   What other choices did I have?
  4.3   What would be the consequences of these other choices?

5 Learning
  5.1   How can I make sense of this experience in light of past experience and future practice?
  5.2   How do I **NOW** feel about this experience?
  5.3   Have I taken effective action to support myself and others as a result of this experience?
  5.4   How has this experience changed my way of knowing in practice?
            Empirics
            Ethics
            Personal
            Aesthetics
  Carper B (1978) Fundamental patterns of knowing in nursing. *Advances in Nursing Science* 1; 13-23

Source: Johns C (1994) Nuances of reflection in *Journal of Clinical Nursing* 3:71-75

Burton (2000)

What......? (This includes a description)

- Is the purpose of returning to this situation?
- Happened?
- Did I see/do?
- Was my reaction to it?
- Did other people do who were involved in this?

So What? (Analysis of the event)

- How did I feel at the time of the event?
- Were those feelings I had any different from those of other people who were involved at the time?
- Are my feelings now, after the event, any different from what I experienced at the time?
- Do I still feel troubled, if so, in what way?
- What are the effects of what I did (or did not do)?
- What positive aspects now emerge for me from the event that happened in practice?
- What have I noticed about my behaviour in practice by taking a more measured look at it?
- What observations does any person helping me to reflect on my practice make of the way I acted at the time?

Now what? (proposed actions following the event)

- What are the implications for me and others in clinical practice based on what I have described and analysed?
- What difference does it make if I chose to do nothing?

- Where can I get more information to face a similar situation?

- How could I modify my practice if a similar situation was to happen again?

- What help do I need to help me 'action' the results of my reflections?

- Which aspect should be tackled first?

- How will I notice that I am any different in clinical practice?

- What is the main learning that I take from reflecting on my practice in this way?

(Source: adapted from Driscoll 2007 page 45)

Iterative models

These include the idea that the reflective process is described as a cycle. The cyclical approach helps you to deepen awareness, increase knowledge and gain appropriate skills through this series of reflections. Gibbs (1988) (figure 3.3) is widely used within health care although other similar models have been developed by Boud et al (1985), Atkins and Murphy (1994) and Blaber (2008). Reid (1993) suggests the use of Gibbs cycle, in conjunction with Goodman's (1984) levels for reflection, is useful to challenge practitioners to think more creatively about the quality of their reflection and a good place to start. Each of these cyclical models follows a similar approach. They start with an experience in the form of a '*critical incident*' or '*learning experience*'. The critical incident is then analysed and evaluated to identify learning, need for further knowledge or demonstrates an understanding of the practice that has taken place. From here an action plan is developed for future practice and the learner can build on the knowledge they have gained from this situation (see Figure 3.3). Unlike the structured model above, this implies a continuous process that develops and continues as you develop in practice.

A worked example of this model can be seen in the last chapter.

Figure 3.3   Gibbs cyclical model of reflection

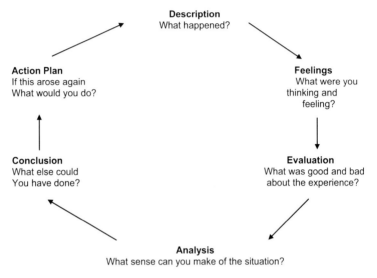

(Gibbs 1988)

Hierarchical models

These models describe different levels of reflection and are based on a hierarchical approach where each step is more complex than the last, resulting in a kind of climbing a ladder approach. Mezirow's (1981) model is an example of this (see Figure 3.4). He uses the ladder approach which goes from describing and identifying the incident, to the 'mastery' of reflection at the final stage of reflection which he refers to as 'theoretical'. There is a prerequisite for moving onto the next level and learning occurs by some inclusion in the levels but only by going through the previous stages.

Other authors that use this approach include Van Manen (1977) and Goodman (1984) although these authors only use three levels of reflection.

Figure 3.4 Mezirow's Seven Levels of Reflection

1. Reflectivity
The act of becoming aware of a specific perception, meaning or behaviour of your own or the habits you have of seeing, thinking and acting.

2. Affective
Becoming aware of how you feel about the way you are perceiving, thinking or   acting.

3. Discriminant
Assessing the efficacy of your perceptions, thoughts and actions. Recognising the reality of the contexts in which you work and identifying your   relationship   to   the   situation.

4. Judgemental
Making and becoming aware of your value judgements, about your perceptions, thoughts and actions, in terms of being positive or negative .

5. Conceptual
Being conscious of your awareness and being critical of it (e.g. being critical of the concepts you use to evaluate a situation).

6. Psychic
Recognising in yourself the habit of making precipitant judgements about people   based   on   limited   information.

7. Theoretical
Becoming aware of the influence of underlying assumptions upon your judgement.

(Mezirow 1981)

Which model to choose?

It does not matter which model you use, or if you choose not to use one at all. A model is a framework to help and guide you when you start to reflect on your practice. By working through them, they can help you to formulate a structured approach to learning and the development of your practice. Again be careful that you do not always reflect on the negative aspects of your practice as we can forget the positive so easily as stated earlier.

Summary

In this chapter we have offered a selection of models. However as stated above, there are many more in the literature. Each one has its own place and you can use one, more than one depending on the situation, or an eclectic approach where you merge models.

In the following chapter we will review some of the uses of reflection and in the final chapter we provide you with some worked examples of reflections using some of the models described in this chapter.

Chapter 4

Learning through, for and from your practice

In this chapter we will identify three areas that relate to learning and your role as a paramedic in practice. These include learning through your practice, learning for your practice and learning from your practice. It will also identify how you can use these three approaches and develop those skills of reflection.

During your training and work you will have experienced different ways of learning. In the classroom, through your personal research and by completing assignments you learn theory related to your practice as a paramedic. This theory is usually taught or evidence based theory through other professional's research.

Other ways you will, or have learnt, is through doing your job. On the job learning by actually having a go, or 'learning from Nellie' that is to say watching someone else do something and learning from their practice through observation. However you learn you need to make sure you are learning the right information and skills in order to carry out your role effectively and safely. Even with reflection you need to make sure that we are learning the right way and improving and developing your practice.

Learning through practice

This learning in practice can be learning-in-action (Schön 1987). Learning and reflecting as you perform and develop your practical skills in the work place.

Not all theory comes through books, research and classroom sessions. You are constantly learning in your workplace and need to take advantage of any experience that you can be involved in or observe.

Some practitioners argue that reflection-in-action is not possible in some situations as there is no time to reflect at the same time as delivering care. There will not always be time when you are faced with an emergency situation to take time out, record or write the reflection. Some people might claim they go onto 'automatic pilot' when faced with these situations. Our argument would be that without thinking you are a dangerous practitioner. Even in the worst situation there is time to draw on your past experiences and reflect on what you did least time or in a similar situation. This thinking might be done instantly and in-the-moment. But thinking and taking check is important at all times. This type of reflection assists you as the paramedic to develop critical thinking in action.

Other times you can take time to reflect whilst you are in your place of work. Learning through practice cannot be found in classroom and your essays; it is through your actual hands-on experience.

The R-Learning cards that were discussed in chapter 2 can help you record short notes of the event, soon after the emergency has passed, so that you can reflect on and analyse it in more detail later.

Learning for practice

Here you learn for your work, what theories support what you are doing and new theories to implement. This learning might be through classroom taught sessions, other training programmes, and through your own research. It may even be through some empirical research that you are personally engaged in. This might also include some learning through trial and error.

Some paramedics might think that once they register then they have learnt all the theory they need for their career. This is not true; at registration you are deemed a competent and safe paramedic. You have a long way to becoming an expert in your field. Reflection is a process that is useful throughout your career and helps you to continually learn for your practice.

Being a paramedic means working in an ever changing environment. As threats of major disasters increase, terrorism or major incidents escalate, you work in an ever-changing environment that you need to constantly keep up to date in and learn for the potential situations. Here we can see some of what we referred to earlier as anticipated reflection (Van Manen 1977).

This learning for practice is also noted in your professional standards as discussed earlier This is why the Health and Care Professions Council, College of Paramedics and Knowledge and Skills Frameworks set out standards to achieve and ask for evidence of your continual learning for your practice.

By constantly reflecting upon and learning from your practice, you can move it forward, developing from and through that practice as noted above.

Learning from practice

We need to learn from what we do as discussed earlier but we can also reflect on what we have done. This is what Schön (1987) refers to as reflection-on-practice. This is when you can take time out after an event or experience. This allows time to critically analyse and evaluate your practice. You can record this at the time by completing the reflective records or writing a piece of reflection.

In this situation you might also review other points of view, relook at your practice through another perspective. How could I have done this differently?

Through this reflection-on-action an action plan is developed for the next time that situation arises. This will help inform your practice rather than just trying to implement another way without first addressing some of the fundamental issues that resulted in that situation.

You might not always record this process formally within a journal or learning log, but the process will help you to become a better paramedic and develop your practice in a systematic way.

Do not forget that you can learn from you work by not only looking at things that did not go well, but also things that went well. This means adopting that appreciative reflection we talked about in the previous chapter.

Learning from practice can also take place in the classroom through the use of narratives and storytelling from your practice (Spouse 2003 and Lillyman et al 2010). This is when you and are able to reflect on the learning in a safe environment and use the tutors expertise, or other colleagues experience, to relate your learning to theory. This is what we referred to earlier in the book as collective wisdom (Ghaye et al 2008) gaining other peoples' inputs.

Processes

The recording of reflection and analysis of significant practice events can facilitate learning. This learning can be of a technical, practical and emancipatory nature. For example:

* '**The technical:** how you as the paramedic practitioner achieves something concrete and instrumental. In this sense you can be seen as a means to clearly specified ends such as gaining recognition of your work and learning within your workplace.

* **The practical:** how reflection facilitates, nourishes and sustains your ability to make wise, competent and ethical decisions and to act compassionately and truly given the clinical context. Examples of this are clarifying the nature of your professional values, engaging in meaningful dialogues with patients and deepening your understanding of the links between practice and theory.

* **The emancipatory:** this is about questioning the status quo, the taken-for-grantedness of our clinical worlds and the historical, social and political forces that serve to liberate and constrain your work. Examples of this are the way the Professional Journal and the analysis of critical incidents generate nursing knowledge and can help to develop you as a critically reflective practitioner.'

(Adapted from Ghaye and Lillyman 2006 pg 103-4)

Outputs and outcomes

When you are reflecting on your practice and working as a reflective practitioner, it is important to appreciate the difference between outputs and outcomes. This is especially important when completing your portfolios and essays. What comes out of the end of a reflective process is an output and the outcome is linked to your performance and achievement.

The output of your reflection can be measured in terms of your learning and recorded within your profile and essays. For example when completing a piece of reflection as an essay or for your portfolio you need to identify what you have learnt and your action plan for the future. These can both be outputs of your reflection. They can be quantified and identified and need to be included within the reflection.

The outcome on the other hand is difficult to measure as the outcome would be 'to be a reflective paramedic'. This is not easy to identify as the process to becoming one is complex, as we have seen earlier in this book.

The outcome will be that you are developing the reflective skills and demonstrating that you are working as a reflective paramedic.

Summary

By using any of the models and approaches described within the book, you can start to move your practice forward in a systematic way. You cannot afford to count the end of your education/training as the end of learning, for the professional paramedic role is constantly evolving and developing and so should you as a professional paramedic. The practice of reflection supports the process of lifelong learning, which is fully supported by the Health and Care Professions Council (2014).

Learning through, for and from practice should be a continual process.

Chapter 5

Examples of using reflective models and approaches

Introduction

In this chapter we provide you with some worked examples of reflection using some of the models and approaches we reviewed in chapter 2.

The following examples are situations, critical incidents, case studies and learning events taken from practice. These might be recorded primarily using the R-Learning Cards and Record Sheets and then developed further as evidence of development for a course, professional body or personal portfolio. Each model is demonstrated by 2 case study examples. All models use the same case as the first example, to show you the individual characteristics of each model. The latter case studies are different and are provided as additional examples.

Using Ghaye et al's (2008) appreciative approach

This approach, as noted earlier, starts with an appreciation of the good and successful aspects of practice, as opposed to a problem solving approach, noted by most of the other models used within the book. Ghaye et al (2008) argue that once we appreciate what we can do, then we can start to identify where we need to change.

Example 1

What's currently working well and why?

I was willing to listen and accept the opinions and understanding of the patient's parents.

What needs changing and how?

My knowledge was poor in relation to this case, the patient's condition and needs.

What are you/we learning and so what do we need to do next?

I have learnt about ALD and its presentation. I still have to find out about the management of patients with ALD who are having a seizure.

Where do you/we go from here and what are the implications for improving your/our future clinical and managerial action and organizational culture/s?

I need to apply the concept of accepting information and knowledge from patients or patient's relatives, to other situations. For this particular case, I have done some research regarding the emergency management of seizures in ALD patients. I will be able to apply this knowledge in future cases. In addition, I can pass this information to other staff members, in order that patients are managed effectively.

Example 2

What's currently working well and why?

The management of the patient was timely and appropriate

What needs changing and how?

More effective assessment of the patient could have flagged up additional problems earlier thus allowing the patient to be treated more quickly. More effective patient assessment is something that I need to address, perhaps by an education course

What are you/we learning and so what do you/we need to do next?

I am learning that a patient assessment is vital to the rapid and effective treatment of a patient's condition, and can assist with prevention of deterioration.
Next, I need to locate and enroll on a course that will assist me to learn the skills that I need for more effective patient assessment.

Where do you/we go from here and what are the implications for improving your/our future clinical and managerial action and organizational culture/s?

Where I go from here: approach the ambulance service education providers and or external providers for example: universities, to ascertain the most appropriate way of obtaining the additional skills I require.

The implications for my future are: additional knowledge and understanding will assist me to assess patients effectively, and with more confidence. Education and understanding will improve my clinical skills, and therefore me as a rounded practitioner. This may lead to further employment opportunities, thus, I can help to improve the organisational culture.

Analysis of this response

In example 1, the student has chosen to reflect on a very positive situation. Example 2 shows a case where there are a few more negative issues to consider.

R-Learning Cards

The next example is that of a student completing an R-Learning Card and Record Sheet in practice. Here the student completes the R-Card as soon as possible after the incident and then shares the reflective notes with a critical friend or mentor later. The incident can be taken further, for an assignment, in the future if needed and appropriate.

R-Card example 1

Date:	Place of incident:
01/01/2015	Patients home

Competency (tick relevant boxes)

ETHICAL PERCEPTIONS ☑
JUDGEMENT ☑

TEAMWORKING ☑ DECISION
MAKING ☑

COMMUNICATION ☑

R-Card Example 2

Date:	Place of incident:
02/01/2015	Patients home

Competency (tick relevant boxes)

ETHICAL PERCEPTIONS ☑
JUDGEMENT ☑

TEAMWORKING ☑ DECISION
MAKING ☑

COMMUNICATION ☑

R-Learning Record Sheet example 1

1. **Event/Incident**: 999 call to an 18yr old male having a seizure. The patient was post-ictal, GCS 9. He had fitted for about 5 minutes, once only. Patient has Adrenoleucodystrophy (ALD), which causes the seizures. Nothing abnormal when compared to other seizures – but his family have been told to call 999 each time.

2. Look at your **EXPERIENCE/MOTIVATION**, what is the most important thing you are learning
It is vital that I take notice of the patient or the parents – especially when they have conditions that I am not familiar with. It was evident, that the patient's parents had considerable knowledge about their son's condition, therefore, it was sensible to be guided by them, unless their decisions appeared to put the patient in danger.

3. Look at your **VALUES/CONFIDENCE**, what is the most important thing you are learning?
Prior to this case, I was reluctant to give the patient or their relatives much say in the management of my patient. This was because I felt that I was the person in charge, and the success or failure of interventions relied upon my decision-making. However, in this case I had virtually no understanding of the patient's condition, so I had little choice in listening to his parents. I found that they were very knowledgeable and were able to provide me with a large amount of information about the patient. This has given me more confidence in listening to the patients and relatives.

4. My **priority for action** is ...
To ensure I listen more to patients and relatives. Learn a little more about ALD.

1. **Event/Incident**: Answered a 999 call to a lady who had fallen with unknown injuries. The lady was on the floor in the hallway, conscious and breathing, although she appeared a little confused (GCS14). She was pale, and did not admit to pain and she had no obvious injuries.

2. Look at your **EXPERIENCE/MOTIVATION**, what is the most important thing you are learning?

I have learnt the importance of gaining a full medical history in order to make a differential diagnosis. The importance of a full head to toe examination which revealed a possible new diagnosis of Atrial Fibrillation (AF).
Also communication skills with the patient and husband who did not want her to go to hospital. Out of hours GP refused to visit as insisted the patient go to hospital.

3. Look at your **VALUES/CONFIDENCE**, what is the most important thing you are learning?
The patient and husband were reluctant to go to hospital and this was not considered further. There was no attempt to discover why there was a fear in relation to admission or the offer of a different hospital.
Conflict in personal values and beliefs in relation to the patient being admitted to hospital.
There was good communication between the crew and patient that was not hurried.

4. My **priority for action** is ...Assessing a patients temperature could have assisted in the request for the patient to go to hospital or in requesting a GP to attend. Finding out why the patient did not want to go to hospital, in order to allay fears, if possible, address issue

REFLECTIVE ADDITIONAL NOTES FOR EXAMPLE 1

Identify what you have learned from your R-Card:

In this incident there was a conflict between my concerns and values. I was able to communicate effectively with most patients and their relatives, however, I was less likely to take seriously their desires and opinions with regards to patient management. In this case, I became very aware of my lack of knowledge, and made a decision to listen and base some decisions on the patient's parents' opinions. The outcome was a positive one for the patient and his parents.

Following discussion what is your agreed action plan:

To give more consideration to patients and relatives opinions. Consider utilizing these opinions in conjunction with my own knowledge, and where necessary with other agencies for example GPs, hospitals.

Following discussion this must be signed by either your mentor/facilitator or tutor:

Signature ………**SMITH**………… Date ……01.01.12……………

REFLECTIVE ADDITIONAL NOTES FOR EXAMPLE 2

Identify what you have learned from your R-Card:

In this incident there was a conflict in my concerns and values. Although there was a good communication between the patient and the crew we did not really explore the patient's reason for not wanting to be admitted. Although we had requested support from the out of hours GP's this was not given leaving the crew to decide on the best possible care for the patient and her husband.

I did feel that clinical decisions were appropriate and that the patient was assessed effectively and thoroughly. Temperature had been taken and therefore could not rule out the possibility of a urinary tract infection (UTI)

Following discussion what is your agreed action plan:

To continue with the head to toe assessment and full history taking.
To rule out possible infections by taking the temperature.
To ascertain if there was other problems in relation to the particular hospital and where possible offer an alternative one.

> **Following discussion this must be signed by either your mentor/facilitator or tutor:**
>
> Signature ... S̶ ̶SMITH ...... Date ....02.01.12...................

Using Johns (2004) structured model of reflection

As noted in the previous chapters, John's model includes a series of cue questions for the practitioner to work through. The first student's example uses all the cue questions.

Example 1 using John's model

---

1. Description

1.1 Write a description of the experience.
Called out following a 999 call to male patient who had suffered a seizure.

1.2 What are the key issues within this description that I need to pay attention to?
Professional practice in relation to decision-making and ethical issues.

---

2. Reflection

2.1 What was I trying to achieve?
Gain a full history and assessment of the patient and appropriate management of the patient.

2.2 Why did I act as I did?
In order to adhere with my professional body and the code of conduct, and to ensure the patient was managed appropriately.

2.3 What are the consequences of my actions?
For the patient and family?
The patient was fully assessed, however, his condition (ALD) was unknown to me. The patient's parents were happy to explain his condition and problems associated with it. I was able to listen and base decisions upon his parent's wishes and hospital advice. My actions ultimately were appropriate for the patient, his family and the service.

For myself?
I am happy with the outcome of this case. I believe that in future, I will be more willing to listen to the opinions of patients and their relatives, basing decisions on them where appropriate.

For the people I work with?
I was working alone when I attended this case, therefore the impact on others is minimal.

2.4 How did I feel about this experience when it was happening?
At the time, I felt uncomfortable as I did not understand the patient's condition and therefore how to treat him effectively. When his parents started to give me information, I felt embarrassed to begin with, but as they explained further, it became clear that they had an excellent understanding of his condition. I therefore decided to find out as much as I could, in order that I could manage the patient appropriately.

2.5 How did the patient feel about it?
The patient was unable to give any opinions due to his condition, however, his parents were very happy with the outcome

2.6 How do I know how the patient felt about it?

The patient was unable to communicate verbally, and had severe mental disability. His parents however, verbally expressed their gratitude and stated that the outcome was the best one for their son.

3. Influencing factors

3.1 What internal factors influenced my decision-making and actions?

Lack of knowledge, desire to ensure I was managing the patient well.

3.2 What external factors influenced my decision-making and actions?

The patient's condition, his parents attitudes and knowledge.

3.3 What sources of knowledge did or should have influenced my decision making and actions?

My own knowledge, the patient's parent's knowledge, hospital consultant.

4. Alternative strategies

4.1 Could I have dealt better with the situation?

No, I believe I acted appropriately.

4.2 What other choices did I have?

I could have insisted the patient attend hospital.

4.3 What would be the consequences of these other choices?

The patient would have been emotionally disturbed, his parent's would have had to get childcare for their other son, an ambulance would have been called and another patient could have had delayed ambulance due to me asking for one.

5. Learning

5.1 How can I make sense of this experience in light of past experience and future practice?
Past experiences have perhaps clouded my opinions of patients and their relatives. In addition, I felt that I should know about all conditions. It is now obvious to me that I cannot understand everything.

5.2 How do I NOW feel about this experience?
I am happy with the way this case went.

5.3 Have I taken effective action to support myself and others as a result of this experience?
Yes.

5.4 How has this experience changed my way of knowing in practice?
It has made me more aware of what I do not know.

Example 2 using John's model

1. Description

1.1 Write a description of the experience.
Called out following a 999 call to male patient who was possibly intoxicated.

1.2 What are the key issues within this description that I need to pay attention to?
Professional practice in relation to decision making and ethical issues.

2. Reflection

2.1 What was I trying to achieve?
Gain a full history and assessment of the patient.

2.2 Why did I act as I did?
In order to adhere with my professional body and the code of conduct, and to ensure the patient was managed appropriately.

2.3 What are the consequences of my actions?
For the patient and family?
The patient was partially assessed, as there were certain procedures he would not agree to, for example blood sugar reading was not consented to. It is unknown how this event would impact upon the patient's family.

For myself?
I am not comfortable that I did not complete an assessment of this patient. This failure could lead to deterioration of the patient's condition, disability or possibly the patient's death. These things could lead to a complaint from the patient or his family, which could result in me losing my HPC registration and therefore my job.
Conversely, there may be no consequences.

For the people I work with?
As I was working with a technician, it is unlikely there will be any consequences for them, apart from taking part in an investigation should a complaint be made. Complaints however, can be stressful for everyone involved, therefore this could be a consequence for my colleague.

2.4 How did I feel about this experience when it was happening?
I felt uncomfortable with this experience, as I was not able to do my job.

2.5 How did the patient feel about it?
I think the patient was angry.

2.6 How do I know how the patient felt about it?
The patient spent a lot of the time shouting at me.

3. Influencing factors

3.1 What internal factors influenced my decision-making and actions?
I was anxious as I have experienced intoxicated patients before, and I was concerned that this man would become aggressive like others have done.

3.2 What external factors influenced my decision-making and actions?
It was cold and dark outside, I didn't want to be out there, and I don't think the patient did either. By trying to get the patient in the ambulance quickly, it also shielded us from other people who may also be intoxicated and potentially violent.

3.3 What sources of knowledge did or should have influenced my decision making and actions?
Experience influenced my decision-making, however, each patient is individual,therefore perhaps, I should not have assumed this patient would be the same as other patients I have experienced.

4. Alternative strategies

4.1 Could I have dealt better with the situation?
Yes definitely.

4.2 What other choices did I have?
I could have taken more time to talk to the patient, explored his history in more detail. I could have let my colleague deal with the patient. I could also have not let my preconceptions cloud my judgment of this patient.

4.3 What would be the consequences of these other choices?

I could have discovered if the shouting was due to the patient being hard of hearing, he may have explained more about his medical history, thus, helping me to understand his needs.

5. Learning

5.1 How can I make sense of this experience in light of past experience and future practice?
Past experiences have impacted upon my behaviour towards this patient. However, experience can aid me, as without it, I may have inadvertently put myself in danger. However, apart from shouting, this patient did not show any signs of aggression, therefore it is likely that he would have remained passive.

5.2 How do I NOW feel about this experience?
I now feel ashamed that I did not treat manage the patient as effectively as I could have. However, I also acknowledge that prior experiences can make me more safety conscious, and therefore these thoughts and feeling should not be ignored.

5.3 Have I taken effective action to support myself and others as a result of this experience?
Yes, I believe that I have.

5.4 How has this experience changed my way of knowing in practice?
I now have a better understanding of the way I think, and why I think and behave the way I do. It will allow me to apply my previous knowledge and experiences in a more appropriate manner – using them as a guide rather than as a definitive answer.

Analysis of this student's reflections

In the both of the examples above the student has systematically worked through the cue questions. However it might be that you only include the subtitles such as:

- Description

- Reflection

- Influencing factors

- Alternative strategies

- Learning

Using Gibbs cyclical model of reflection

The following incidents are taken from events that happened following 999 calls. They are written from the student's perspective.

Example 1: Using Gibb's model (1988)

Describing the incident

I was working as a solo responder, and I received a 999 call to an 18 year old male patient who was having a seizure. On arrival, I was greeted by the patients' parents. They told me that the patient had adrenoleukodystrophy (ALD), which I was not familiar with.

The patient had stopped seizing, but was not fully conscious. I assessed the patient fully, and found nothing abnormal apart from his GCS. After waiting for half an hour with the patient and his family, the patient had recovered and was his normal self. His GCS was still very low, as according to his parents, the patient had a mental age of 3. After a conversation with the patient's consultant, it was felt appropriate to leave the him in the care of his family. I advised his parents that they should call 999 again if they were worried or if the patient should have another seizure.

Feelings

En route, I felt quite confident as I have dealt with patients having seizures previously and I knew what I could be faced with. However, on arrival, I felt quite uncomfortable as I was completely unaware of the patient's medical condition and the consequences of it. The patient's
parents were very understanding as their sons condition was quite rare, and therefore, they did not expect me to know about it. I became more at ease as the patient's parents explained his condition, and became quite sympathetic to their experiences. On leaving the address, I was quite happy that the management applied was appropriate and supportive for both patient and his family. Looking back on the event now, I am happy that what I did was right, and I am grateful that the patient's family were willing to provide information and assist with my understanding of the patient's condition.

Evaluation

The good points were, although the patient's underlying medical condition was unknown to me, I understood what I needed to do with patients' who were having seizures. Having a good understanding of the JRCALC guidelines (Fisher et al 2006) and my local protocols and guidelines gave me confidence in managing the patient's seizures. Once I recognised my lack of knowledge of ALD could have serious consequences for the patient, I asked the patient's parents to explain his condition to me. The patient's parents showed a great deal of understanding and were very happy to explain everything they knew about their son's condition. I was receptive to their knowledge and understanding.

The negatives were that I did not understand the patient's condition and therefore if there was anything more I could have done. Nor did I know if any of the treatments I could have used would have been detrimental to the patient's condition.

Analysis

The Health and Care Professions Council (2014) state that paramedics should always act in the patients best interest and within the confines of legislation. I worked within Fisher et al's (2006) guidelines for the management of patients including patient's having seizures, which includes best practice and current legislation. The Health and Care Professions Council (2014) state that communication with service users is a vital part of any paramedics practice. I was able to communicate very effectively with my patients parents, who were able to provide me with a great deal of information regarding the patient's underlying medical condition. Booker (2005) recommends showing respect for the patient's opinions, and to continually develop one's own knowledge. I believe in this case I did both of these, although the patient did not have an opinion that he could demonstrate, therefore, I utilised his parents' viewpoint and opinions instead. Having no knowledge of ALD prior to this incident, I was also able to develop my own knowledge as Booker (2005) suggests. Booker also advises that the most effective decisions are made in collaboration with service users; again this is something that I was able to do.

In terms of the negative aspects, I realise that it is not possible for me to know about every condition, especially the more unusual ones. In this case, had it been likely that there would adverse reactions from my management techniques, the patients family would have been informed by their consultant.

Conclusion

In response to what else could I have done: I could have been more willing to ask the patients family about his condition early on in the case. I could have insisted the patient and his family attend hospital, especially as I was unfamiliar with any potential problems resulting from the seizure. I do not believe that this course of action would have been beneficial, as the patient's family were familiar with his condition, and were happy to look after him. In addition, they knew that they could use the 999 system again if necessary.

I could have insisted that the patient's GP visit the patient, however he was not familiar with the patient's condition (as the patient was managed by a hospital consultant).

I could have left prior to the recovery of the patient, however, to do so could be problematic if the patient has started seizing again – thus delaying treatment.

I could have not called the patients consultant, which would have left me not knowing the best course of action for this patient and his family.

Action plan

If I encounter the same case again, I would again communicate with the patient's family and take their wishes into account, however in future I would hope to be more open to this earlier on within the management of the patient.

References

Booker R (2005) Effective Communication with the Patient. *European Respiratory Review.* Vol 14, No 96, pp.93-96.

Fisher, J., Brown, N. and Cooke, M. (2006) UK Ambulance service guidelines. Warwick: Ambulance Service Association.

Health and Care Professions Council (2014) *Standard of Proficiency: Paramedics.* Health and Care Professions Council: London.

Health and Care Council (2014) *Standards of Conduct, Performance and Ethics.* Health and Care Council: London.

Example 2: Using Gibb's model

Describing the incident
I was working as part of a crew, we were called to a 85 year old lady who had fallen whilst trying to get to the toilet. We discovered that she was uninjured. I assessed the patient and found nothing out of the ordinary. We lifted the patient back into her chair, and left her at home. Another ambulance was called to this same patient later that day, and she was admitted to hospital for a UTI.

Feelings
En route, I did not experience any particular emotion, as I have attended many cases of this type. On arrival, I felt sad for the patient, as she was upset at being on the floor for quite a while. I also felt sad that the patient was alone at home, her husband having died recently. After the case I felt quite happy that I had done the right thing, however, when I discovered the patient had been admitted later in the day, I felt very guilty that I had missed the UTI.

Evaluation
There are both positive and negative points within this case. I dealt with the initial issue of the fall with compassion and gave the patient some dignity. I communicated effectively with the patient, however, I failed to consider UTI, therefore did not ask pertinent questions or consider referral to her GP.

Analysis
The Health Professions Council (2007) state that paramedics should always act in the patient's best interest and within the confines of legislation. I worked within ambulance service guidelines with regards to the fall. The Health Professions Council (2008) state that communication with service users is a vital part of any paramedics practice. I was able to communicate effectively with my patient, and assess her appropriately for injuries. Caroline (2009) advocates good patient assessment, in order to prevent injuries or conditions being missed. I believe that I did not fully assess this patient, as I failed to ask her about urinary habits/problems.

Conclusion
I could have asked the patient about any urinary problems and completed a further assessment. I could have contacted a relative of the patient. I could have requested a GP to visit the patient, or I could have requested that the patient attend hospital.

Action plan
If I encounter the same case again, I consider further assessment with UTI in mind, I will consider requesting a GP visit – if that cannot be arranged, I will consider asking the patient to attend hospital – explaining why.

References
Caroline N (2009) *Emergency Care in the Streets.* (6th Ed) Jones and Bartlett: London.

Health and care Professions Council (2014) *Standard of Proficiency: Paramedics.* Health Professions Council: London.

Health and Care Professions Council (2014) *Standards of Conduct, Performance and Ethics. Health* Professions Council: London.

Reflection using an eclectic approach

We can take the principles of the models discussed in chapter 3 and record your reflections as suits your style. Below we have given some further examples developed from the published models.

Example 1: Using an eclectic model

Description of incident/event

I was working as a solo responder, and I received a 999 call to an 18 year old male patient who was having a seizure. On arrival, I was greeted by the patients' parents. They told me that the patient had adrenoleukodystrophy (ALD), which I was not familiar with.

The patient had stopped seizing, but was not fully conscious. I assessed the patient fully, and found nothing abnormal apart from his GCS. After waiting for half an hour with the patient and his family, the patient had recovered and was his normal self. His GCS was still very low, as according to his parents, the patient had a mental age of 3. After a conversation with the patient's consultant, it was felt appropriate to leave the him in the care of his family. I advised his parents that they should call 999 again if they were worried or if the patient should have another seizure.

By whom was it handled?

I handled the whole case.

What learning experiences occurred?

I learnt a great deal about ALD which I did not know. I also learnt that I am not expected to know everything about every condition.

What were the outcomes of this incident?

The outcomes of the incident were all positive. The patient was manage appropriately to prevent further deterioration of his condition. I had a learning experience which has allowed me to develop and grow as a practitioner.

How has this incident affected your practice?

This incident has given me knowledge which I can apply to other similar situations or patients with the same conditions. In addition, it has given me the confidence to acknowledge that I am not familiar with all medical conditions and ask patients or their relatives for information.

Example 2: Using an eclectic model

Description of Incident/event
Whilst working with an ambulance technician, I was called out to a male patient who was reported to be intoxicated.

By whom was it handled?
I had most contact with the patient in this case.

What learning experiences occurred?
I learnt that I should let my experiences guide but not influence unduly my reactions and behaviour towards a patient.

What were the outcomes of this incident?
The outcomes were that the patient was not fully assessed. This may have been the outcome, regardless of my influences; however, it is possible that the patient would have allowed a full assessment had my behaviour been different.

How has this incident affected your practice?
In future when dealing with similar patients, I will use my experiences to guide me, however, I will also treat each patient as an individual. I will complete a full assessment on each patient regardless of their intoxication level.

Example 3: using an eclectic model

Describing the event
As part of a crew I attended an elderly female patient who had fallen from her bed. She was complaining of pain in her left hip. Upon examination, there was obvious shortening and rotation of the leg. After administering pain relief, we moved the patient onto the stretcher and transported her to hospital. She became very agitated and upset en route to the hospital. Subsequently as we arrived at the hospital, I discovered that her husband had died at the hospital we were going to, which frightened the lady.

By whom was it handled?
My crewmate and myself dealt with this case, I was attending so I had the most contact with the patient.

What learning experiences occurred?
I realised after finding out about the lady's husband that I had not told the patient where we wanted to take her, and we had not asked for consent to do so. Had I done this, it is likely that the patient would have requested transportation to a different hospital (which would have been possible). I had assumed that that the patient knew the most local hospital did not accept trauma patients, therefore I assumed she knew she needed to go to the next most local unit. The lady was unaware of this situation.

What were the outcomes of this incident?
The main outcome was that the patient was emotionally upset by transportation to the hospital. Whilst she undoubtedly needed to attend hospital, and did not refuse transportation, it is possible that the emotional upset that I unwittingly caused this patient may delay her recovery.

How has this incident affected your practice?
I am now more aware of informing patients of my intended actions (where possible). I am also more willing to transport the patient to their hospital of choice, where their condition and logistics allow. Where it is not possible to transport the patient to their chosen hospital, I will explain the reasons for this and give the alternative options (where the patients' condition and logistics allow).

Summary

We have provided you with a variety of incidents and events from practice that can be used for reflection. These will give you some idea of how to record and move your practice on in order to develop to what Benner (1984) describes as the expert practitioner.

Overall Conclusion

Where to from here?

Through reflection you can develop professional skills that are required in order to become an expert paramedic.

Reflection should be part of your everyday practice and when required to be in written format as evidence for assignments, portfolios and personal development plans.

As practice changes so should you. To remain static will result in you becoming out of date and in time a dangerous practitioner.

Reflection and the skill of being a professional practitioner will be valuable for you as a professional, for your patients to improve the quality of service they receive, your colleagues and other students as a knowledgeable practitioner, to the profession as maintaining standards and to your employer as an improver of practice.

This book has provided you with an introduction to reflection and becoming a reflective practitioner. There are many articles and much research completed on this subject.

We wish you well with your reflection and in becoming an expert reflective paramedic.

References

Argyris, M. and Schön D. (1974) *Theory in practice. Increasing professional effectiveness.* San Francisco: Jossey Bass.

Atkins, S., and Murphy, K. (1994) Reflective Practice, Nursing *Standard,* Vol. 8, No. 39, pp. 49-56.

Benner, P. (1984) *From Novice to Expert. Excellence and power in clinical nursing practice.* Commemorative edition. Menlo Park, London: Addison Wesley.

Blaber, A. (2008) *Foundations for Paramedic Practice: A Theoretical Perspective.* Milton Keynes: Open University Press.

Booker R (2005) Effective Communication with the Patient. *European Respiratory Review.* 14 (96) pp.93-96.

Boud, D., Keough, R. *and* Walker, D. (1985) *Reflection: Turning Experience into Learning.* London: Kogan Page.

Bulman, C. & Schutz, S. (2004) *Reflective Practice in Nursing* (eds). (3rd ed). Oxford: Blackwell Publishing Ltd.

Burton, A.J. (2000) Reflection: Nursing's practice and education panacea? *Journal of Advanced Nursing* 31 (5) 1009-1017.

Carper, B. (1978) Fundamental patterns of knowing in nursing. *Advances in Nursing Science* 1(1): 13 – 23.

Caroline, N. (2009) *Emergency Care in the Streets.* (6th Ed) London: Jones and Bartlett.

Chafee, J. (1994) Teaching for critical thinking. *Education Vision* 2(1) 24-25.

Chene, A. (1983) *The concept of autonomy: Philosophical discussion* cited in Memarian, S. & Caffarella, R. (eds) *Learning in adulthood*, San Francisco CA: Jossey-Bass Publishers p 215.

College of Paramedics (2015) *CPD Guidance. At* https://www.collegeofparamedics.co.uk/publications/professional-standards

Conceicao, S. and Taylor, L. (2007) Using a constructivist approach with online concept maps: Relationship between theory and nursing education. *Nurse Education in Perspectives* 28(5) 268-275.

Cooney, A. (1999) Reflection demystified: answering some common Questions. *British Journal of Nursing (8)* 22 pp1530-1534.

Department of Health (2004) Knowledge and Skills Framework (NHS KSF) and development review process. London: Department of Health.
.
Dewey, J. (1933) *How we think.* Chicago: Henrey Regney.

Driscoll, J. (2007) *Supported reflective learning: the essence of clinical supervision* in Driscoll, J. (2nd ed) Practicing clinical supervision: A reflective account for health care professionals. Philadelphia: Elsevier.

Facione, N. C. & Facione, P. A. (1996) Externalising the critical thinking in knowledge development and clinical judgement. *Nursing Outlook* 44 pp 129-36.

Finger. M. and Asun. M (2000) *Adult education at the crossroads. Learning our way out.* London: Zed Books.

Fischer, G. & Scharff, E. (1998) learning technologies in support of self directed learning. *Journal of interactive media in Education* 98(4) pp1-28.

Fisher, J., Brown, N. and Cooke, M. (2006) UK Ambulance service guidelines. Warwick: Ambulance Service Association.

Flannagan, J. (1954) The critical incident technique. *Psychological Bulletin*, 51, 327–58.

Germann P and Young-soo. K (2001) Heightening Reflection through Dialogue: A case for electronic journaling and electronic concept mapping in science classes. *Contemporary issues in Technology and Teacher Education* 1(3) 321-333.

Gelter, H. (2003) Why is reflective thinking uncommon? *Reflective Practice* 4 (3) 337-344.

Ghaye, T. & Lillyman, S. (2006) *Learning journals & critical incidents. Reflective practice for health care professionals.*2nd edition, Dinton: Quay Books - Mark Allen.

Ghaye T., Melander-Wikman,A., Kisare, M., Chambers,P., Ulrika, B., Kostenius, C., Lillyman, S. (2008) Participatory and appreciative action and reflection (PAAR) democratizing reflective practices. *Reflective Practice* 9 (4), 361- 398.

Gibbs, G. (1988) *Learning by Doing: A guide to Teaching Learning Methods.* Oxford Polytechnical.

Goodman, J. (1984) Reflection and teacher education. *A case study and theoretical analysis interchange*, 15(3) 9-26 in Rideout, E. (2001). *Transforming Nursing Education through Problem-Based learning.* London; United Kingdom. Jones & Bartlett publishers international.

Haddock, J. (1997) Nurses' perceptions of reflective practice. *Nursing Standard* 11(32):9-41.

Health and Care Professions Council (2014) *Continuing professional development and your registration.* London. Health and Care Professions Council.

Health and Care Professions Council (2015) *Important Dates* at http://www.hpc-uk.org/registrants/cpd/dates/

Health Professions Council (2008) *Standards of Conduct, Performance and Ethics. Health and Care* Professions Council: London.

Health Professions Council (2007) *Standard of Proficiency: Paramedics. London:* Health Professions Council.

Jarvis, P. (1992) Reflective practice and nursing. *Nurse Education Today*, 12, 174-81.

Johns, C., (1994) Nuances of Reflection. *Journal of Clinical Nursing*, 3, pp. 71-75.

Johns, C. (2004) Becoming a Reflective Practitioner (2nd ed.) London: Blackwell Science.

Johns, C. (2006) *Engaging reflection in practice. A narrative approach.* Oxford. Blackwell Publishing Company.

Kim, D. and Lee, S. (2002) Designing collaborative Reflection supporting tools in E-project-based learning environments. *Journal of Interactive learning 13 (4) at www.aace.org/pubs.*

Kolb, D., (1984) *Experiential Learning: Experience as the Source of Learning and Development,* NJ: Prentice Hall.

Lake, A. (2001) *developing personal, social and moral education through physical education. A practical guide for teachers.* Lonond: Routledge Falmer.

Lillyman, S. Gutteridge, R. Berridge. P (2011) Using a storyboarding technique in the classroom to address end of life experiences in practice and engage student nurses in deeper reflection. *Nurse Education in Practice.* 11(3), 179-185

Mezirow, J. (1981) A Critical Theory of Adult Learning and Education. *Adult Education* 32: (1) pp 3-24.

Newell, R. (1992) Anxiety, accuracy and reflection: the limits of professional development. *Journal of Advanced Nursing* 17:1326-33.

Powell, J. H. (1989) The reflective practitioner in nursing. *Journal of Advanced Nursing* 14, 824 – 832.

Quinn, F. M. & Hughes, S. J. (2007) *Quinn's Principles and practice of Nurse Education.* 5th edition. United Kingdom: Nelson Thornes, Ltd.

Ramnarayan, K. & Hande, S. (2005) *thoughts on self directed learning in medical schools: making student more responsible. New horizon for learning.* [online] http//:www.newhorisons.org.lifelong

Reid, B (1993) 'But we're Doing It Already!' Exploring a response to the concept of reflective practice in order to improve its facilitation. *Nurse Education Today* (13) 305-309.

Rubenfeld, M. G. & Scheffer, B. K. (1999) *critical thinking in nursing. An interactive approach* (2nd ed) London: Lippincott.

Schön, D. (1973) *Beyond the state. Public and private learning in a changing society.* Harmondsworth: Penguin.

Schön, D. (1983) *The reflective practitioner.* New York: Basic Books.
Schön, D. (1987) *Educating the Reflective Practitioner.* San Francisco: Josey Bass.

Simpson, E. & Courtney, M. (2000) Critical thinking in nursing education: A literature review cited in Turner, C. A. (2000) critical thinking: beyond nursing process. *Journal of Nursing Education* 39(8) 333-339.

Smyth, J. (1991) *Teachers as Collaborative Learners.* Milton Keynes: Open University Press.

Spouse, J. (2003) *Professional Learning in Nursing.* Oxford, Blackwell Publishers.

Taylor, B. J. (2006) *reflective practice. A guide for nurses and midwives.* (2nd ed). Milton Keynes: Open University Press.

Tripp, D. (1993) *Critical Incidents in Teaching.* London: Routledge.
Van Manen, M. (1977) Linking ways of knowing with ways of being practical. *Curriculum Enquiry* 6(3) 205-28.

Yahiro, K. M. & Saylor, C. (1994) A critical thinking model for nursing judgement. *Journal of Nursing Education*, 33(8) 351 – 356.